I'm Not Weird, I Have Sensory Processing Disorder (SPD): Alexandra's Journey

2nd Edition

✳✳✳

by Chynna T. Laird

Loving Healing Press

From the Growing With Love Series at Loving Healing Press.
Visit the author online at www.LilyWolfWords.ca

Library of Congress Cataloging-in-Publication Data

Laird, Chynna T., 1970-
I'm not weird, I have sensory processing disorder (SPD) : Alexandra's journey / by Chynna T. Laird.
-- 2nd ed.
p. cm. -- (Growing with love series)
Audience: 5-8.
Audience: K to grade 3.
ISBN 978-1-61599-158-7 (pbk.: alk. paper) -- ISBN 978-1-61599-159-4 (hardcover: alk. paper)
-- ISBN 978-1-61599-160-0 (ebook)
1. Sensory integration dysfunction in children--Juvenile literature. 2. Sensory disorders in children
--Juvenile literature. I. Title.
RJ496.S44L34 2012
618.92'8--dc23
2012009882

Distributed by Ingram Book Group (USA/CAN), New Leaf Distributing, Bertram's Books (EU), and
Hachette Livre (FR).

Published by
Loving Healing Press Inc.   www.LHPress.com
5145 Pontiac Trail   info@LHPress.com
Ann Arbor, MI 48105

Tollfree USA/CAN: 888-761-6268
London, UK: 44-20-331-81304

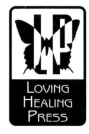

LOVING
HEALING
PRESS

To: Jaimie – my miracle girl

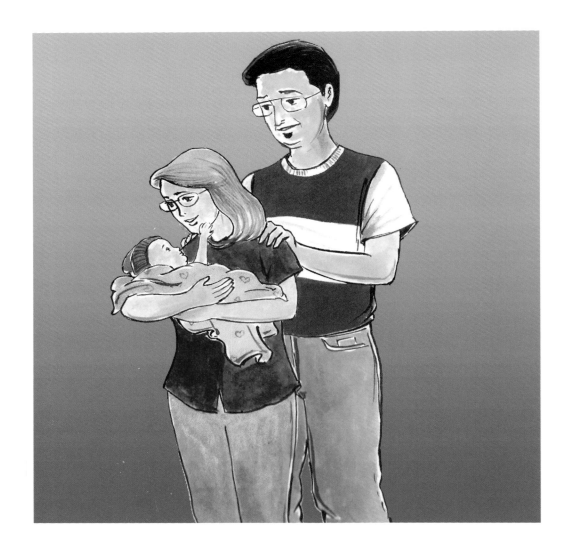

When I was born, I loved everything around me. I liked looking at my Mama and Daddy, I liked hearing their voices, and I loved feeling their arms around me when I needed a cuddle.

But things changed as I grew. Things got scary. So scary, I screamed. It frustrated me because nobody else seemed to feel the scary things I did and it made me mad.

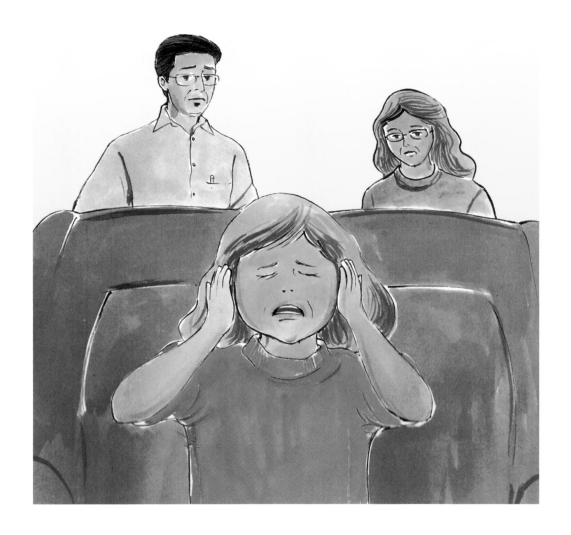

Noises, even whispers, hurt my ears. This made Daddy sad because his voice hurt my ears a lot and I wouldn't let him talk to me. When things got too loud, I covered my ears and screamed until the noises stopped.

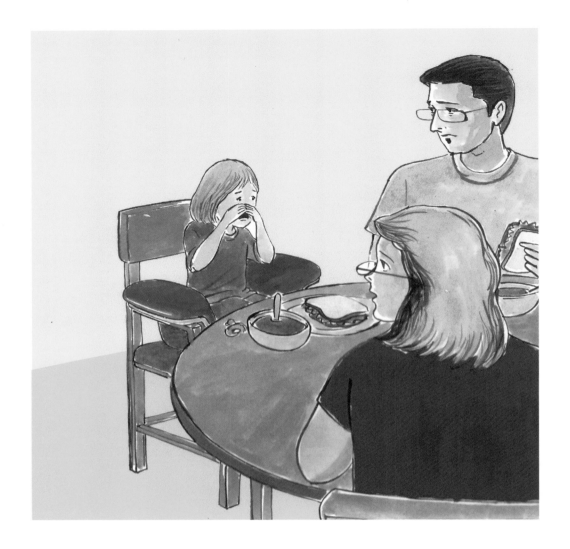

Smells bothered my nose and sometimes made me sick. I smelled things differently than other people did and I also smelled things no one else could. I tried covering my nose but that never worked very well. So I screamed to make the smells go away.

Sometimes when things didn't smell good to me, I wouldn't eat. I thought the yucky smells in my nose were what Mama put on my plate. I tried eating the food anyway but if it didn't feel good on my tongue, I got sick. Mama and Daddy couldn't understand why the food I used to eat starting upsetting me so much.

6

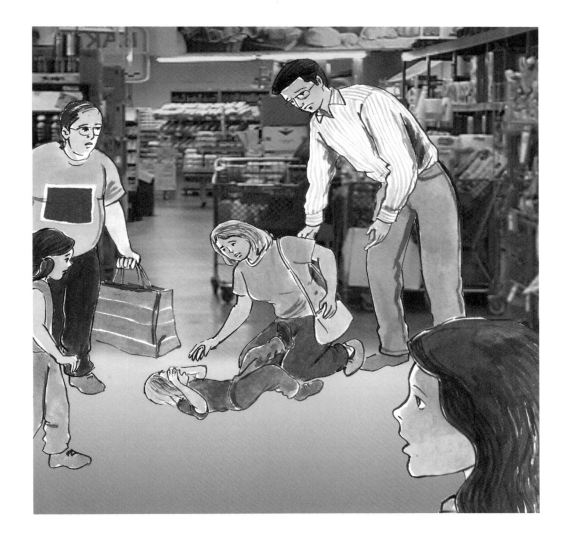

The lights in stores or in other people's houses hurt my eyes. My eyes hurt even more when I went outside on a bright, sunny day. I covered my eyes to block out the brightness and screamed to make the pain stop.

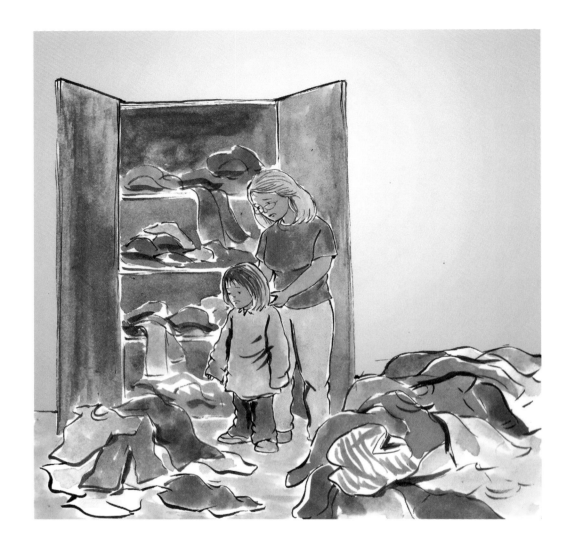

I especially didn't like how things felt on my skin. When the wind blew on my arms and legs, it felt like thousands of creepy caterpillars crawling on me that I couldn't get off. The tags in my clothes tickled me and made me mad so I got Mama to cut all the tags out of my clothes. Sometimes Mama got frustrated with me because I tried on lots of different clothes until something felt just right.

Chynna T. Laird

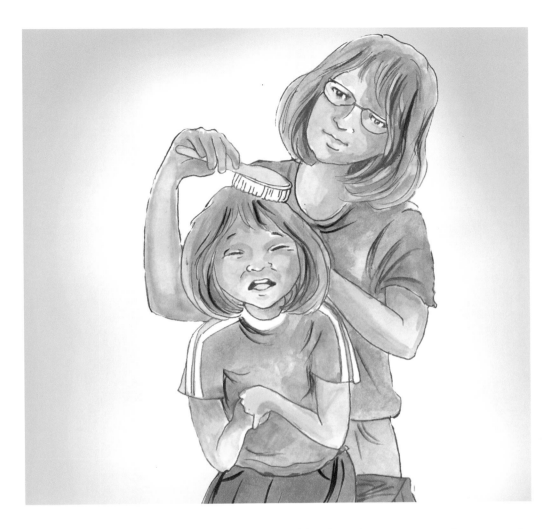

I didn't like the feeling of lots of things and it could be hard getting ready some days. Brushing my teeth made me gag; brushing my hair hurt so bad, I cried or hid from Mama; bath time was scary because the water tickled my skin and if it was too hot or cold, it hurt me; and I hated my winter clothes.

Everything had to be the same. I liked my bed and bedroom to be the same way. I liked knowing what we were going to do because when things changed, it was too confusing for me. When things were the same, I felt safe. When things were different or changed or there were too many things to remember, I got scared and cried.

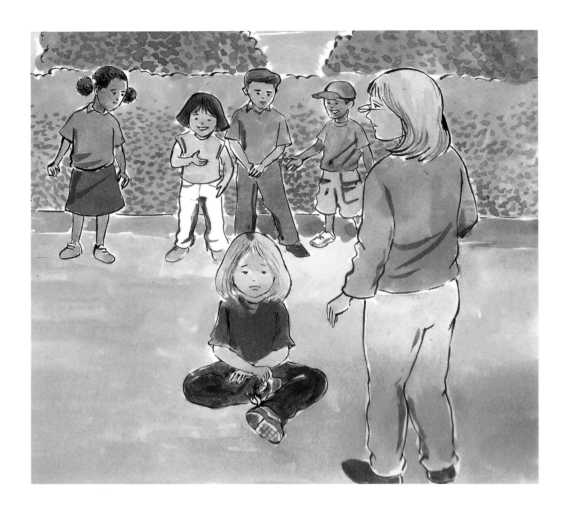

Touch scared me a lot. I didn't like people touching me and I didn't know how to tell people their fingers felt like fire on my skin. Mama and Daddy wanted to hug me but I couldn't let them.

I fell down a lot too. My arms, legs, hands and feet didn't always listen to what my head told them to do. Sometimes when I tried doing stuff, my body got all tangled up and I ended up crashing down on the ground. It didn't always hurt, though.

At the park, I didn't like playing the same games the other kids played. They liked climbing high or sliding or going down the poles or swinging and it made my tummy jump doing that stuff. One time, I climbed the ladders but couldn't remember how to get back down. Then I was too scared to climb anymore or even let someone lift me up.

Chynna T. Laird

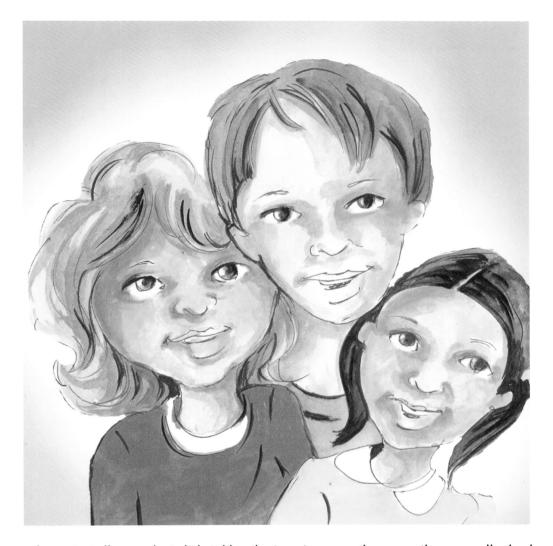

I didn't know how to tell people I didn't like their voices; or the way they smelled when they got too close; or the way their faces moved or looked when they talked to me. I didn't know how to tell people I liked them but they scared me.

So I screamed. I screamed long and loud to block out the things that nobody else saw, heard or smelled but me. I even tried hitting my head, scratching my arms, or biting myself to make it all stop—but it never worked.

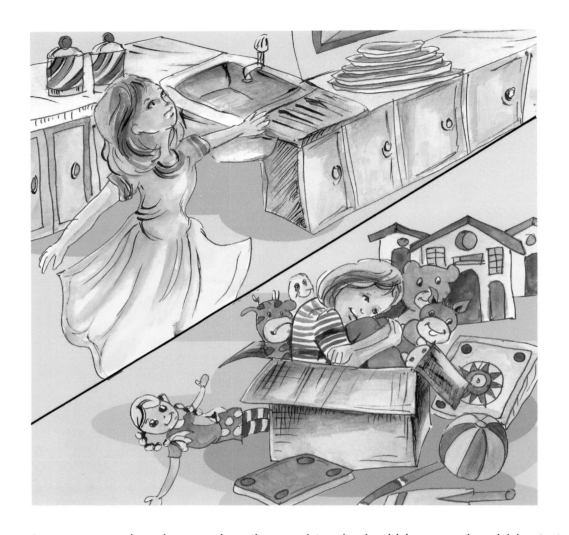

Sometimes I spun around and around until everything looked blurry and wobbly. Or I squeezed myself into tight places, like between the wall and the couch or the snuggly place in my closet or in the stuffy toy box. I never got dizzy when I spun and my body felt safer when I squeezed it. I just didn't know how to tell Mama or Daddy or anyone else that those things made me feel better.

Because I couldn't tell people what was happening to me, or what I wanted to feel better, they thought I was weird especially other children. And some of them even made fun of me. I wanted to explain to them so they understood me but I didn't know how.

Chynna T. Laird

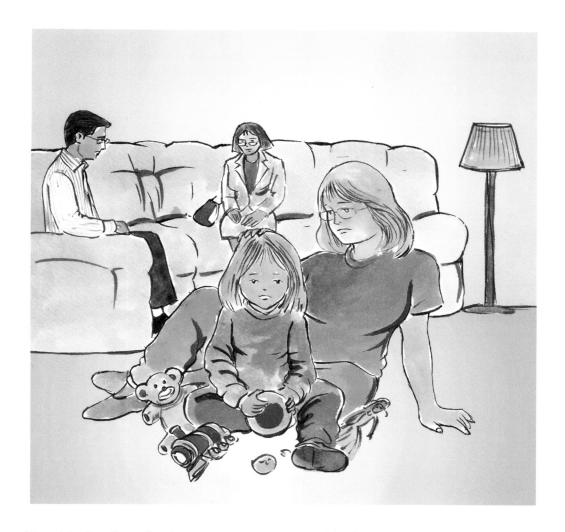

Mama and Daddy finally asked a visitor to come and help us. Her name was Donna and Mama called her an Occupational Therapist. Donna told Mama I had Sensory Processing Disorder. She said it was a mouthful so we could call it SPD for short.

Donna said the reason I got upset all the time was because my brain didn't process things the same way everyone's brain did. She said when I smelled something or felt someone touch me, my brain got the message but it didn't understand how to read it. My brain jumbled up the messages it received and got confused. And when it got confused it got scared and **that's** why I screamed.

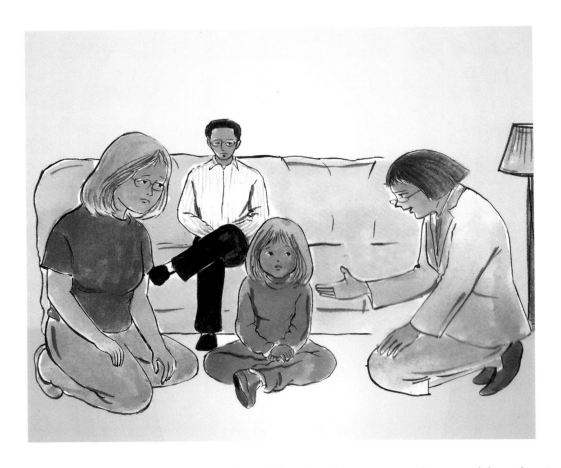

Donna taught me how to tell Mama and Daddy what hurt me so they could understand and she taught Mama and Daddy how to help me use words and gestures to let them know how I felt.

Donna taught me different ways to calm my insides down so I wouldn't scream anymore.

Donna said, "You won't hurt Mama or Daddy's feelings by telling them you don't like hugs, Alexandra. They want you to be happy. They would be sad if they knew their hugs hurt you but you didn't say so."

I'm six now and much bigger. Things still hurt me but I try to use my voice to tell people what's going on inside me instead of screaming. And I use different ways to calm my insides down, like squeezing PlayDoh, swinging, jumping on my trampoline, or putting something heavy on my lap so I won't hurt myself or anyone else.

Chynna T. Laird

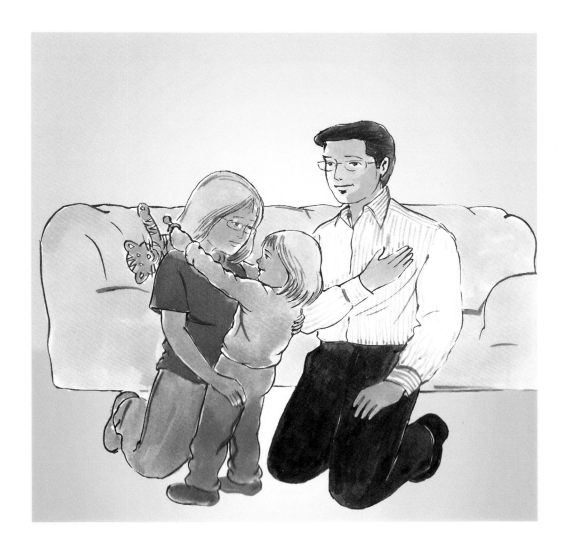

Now whenever we go somewhere, I take my big blue pacifier, named Soodee to block out yucky smells, my beanie Tigger to hug so I felt safe and I wear my beautiful pink sunglasses to stop bright lights and the sun from hurting my eyes. And I'm not afraid to tell people when I don't like them touching or hugging me.

Guess what? I even let myself give Mama a hug a few months ago **for the very first time**! It didn't hurt as much as I thought it would. I don't do it very much but at least I know I **can** do it and Mama will let me hug her again if I want to.

I'm Not Weird, I Have SPD

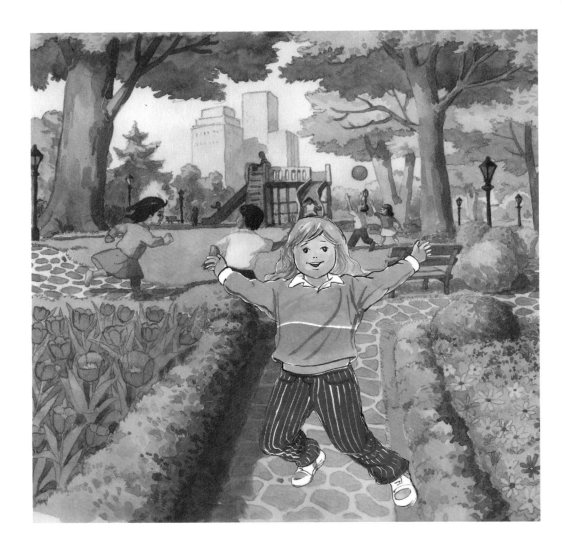

Yes, things are getting better. I know I'll always have SPD but it doesn't scare me as much anymore. Now when other people or kids ask about me or make fun of me, I just tell them: "I'm not weird. I'm Alexandra and I have SPD."

Chynna T. Laird

Sensational Activities

When we took this book to Jaimie's school in Kindergarten, we found that her classmates were very enthusiastic to learn about SPD and how it feels to Jaimie. So we came up with a few suggestions for interactive activities teachers and/or caregivers can do with children while reading along with the story or to try after a reading for discussion.

For more activity suggestions, please contact
Chynna through her website at www.lilywolfwords.ca.

(1) We all react to different kinds of sensory stimulation in different ways. Put together an awareness box filled with different textured objects such as feathers, kooshie balls, slime, sandpaper, etc. Have the children talk about how these objects feel to them and how they might feel to kids like Alexandra.

(2) Children with SPD can also have balance and coordination problems that can interfere with how they play and interact with their peers at recess or gym time. Have readers try activities such as: putting their shoes on the wrong feet and walking around; writing with the opposite hand; bouncing a ball on a rough or uneven surface; spinning around until they're dizzy then trying to walk straight; putting a wooly sweater or similarly "itchy" type of fabric on and trying to concentrate on something else; wearing heavy, warm clothes when it's hot outside; trying to see with very bright lights shining in their faces; have different smelling items or scratch-and-sniff stickers (nice and stinky smells); putting hands in icy cold water—with then without something that would protect their hands from feeling the coldness. (Activities such as the last suggestion are to show that some children with SPD aren't overresponsive but underresponsive and don't feel sensations at all or are slow to react to them.) Then talk about how these activities made them feel and why such things may be difficult and/or frustrating for children with sensory issues. Also talk about how it can be dangerous *not* to feel sensations (such as with the icy water activity).

(3) Ask interactive questions while reading the book such as, "What sorts of clothes make you uncomfortable?" "Here, try pretending there are creepy caterpillars on your skin. How do you think that would feel?" "How do you think we can we help someone like Alexandra show us how to help her feel better?" "What sorts of fun games can we think of that Alexandra would like to play with us?" These help children think about situations from the other child's perspective and learn how to reach out and be reached out to.

(4) Have a Sensational Awareness Week or something similarly themed where you discuss the different senses and how they help us learn about our world and the people in it. Highlight one sensory system each day and include the systems not usually thought of, such as the proprioceptive and vestibular systems (these help us with movement, balance, coordination and discovering our relation to object in our environment.) Be sure to talk about how some people have issues with their senses and discuss how these issues can change how they learn about their own worlds. (October is National Sensory Awareness Month. You could always contact the SPD Foundation at www.spdfoundation.net or S.I. Focus at www.sifocus.com for other ways to help educate children on the senses and SPD.)

(5) Get kids moving with different activities that help to coordinate their bodies, strengthen their balance while also giving them chances to learn through sensory stimulation. Include music time, such as singing songs with movements; have children roll around in the grass; do clay projects where they get to squish and manipulate things and get their hands dirty; give them chances to push/pull/drag objects— games like tug-of-war or playing with medicine balls; have relay races like working a ball with a hockey stick around pile-ons; do wheelbarrow walks or crab-walks. The whole point is to help children become aware of their bodies and what all the parts of their bodies need do *together* to run properly. Children with SPD do a lot of these activities in their occupational therapy (OT) so having these activities at school too gives them extra movement time, which they need. And doing them with friends can make it even more fun!

A final note: It's a good idea to watch children with your "sensory glasses" on to be sure none of these activities cause distress. Encouragement for what steps they can do—not whether they complete everything—is the key.

Chynna T. Laird

Questions For Dr. Lucy Jane Miller

Chynna had the amazing opportunity to chat with Dr. Lucy Miller during Sensory Awareness Month 2011. Dr. Miller's words were so inspirational, Chynna felt compelled to share them here with her readers. You can read the full interview on http://tinyurl.com/spd2012, which includes some of Dr. Miller's advice on how you can raise awareness for SPD.

Here are Dr. Miller's words on:

Her background: It's funny how where I am now, directing the STAR Center in Denver has all grown from seeds planted over 35 years! I started as an Occupational Therapist with a sensory integration therapy frame of reference in Head Start and in an Early Childhood Program, consulting and working with the teachers in the classrooms and doing home visits for children birth to three. My goodness that was a long time ago! Even then I was asking questions and making trouble for those happy with the status quo! It was on my opinion that children were put into the "special education" Head Start classrooms. I was using a test but over time I saw that the test was very inaccurate. That's when I started to develop the Miller Assessment for Preschoolers (MAP), which turned into my first nationally standardized test for children. (Now I have authored 9 norm-referenced standardized scales.) That was 35 years ago, and the rest is a long (and to me interesting journey) but perhaps best left for a radio interview (or a novel!).

On training with Dr. Jean Ayres: Dr. Ayres was a brilliant scholar, a gifted clinician, and a role model for research. She taught me many things but the most important was this: Question everything and everyone. Never believe what you read. Read down into what you read to make sure it is reliable and valid. Ask questions. She said, "Question me, Lucy and question yourself. If you can't ask questions, you'll never be a researcher." I'm very proud that my certification # is 10!

What 'sensational' parents need to know: Parents and other caregivers need to trust their instincts. If they think something is "wrong" with their child, they are probably right. Don't accept what a professional tells you if you know it isn't right. Get a second opinion. Make sure you know what you are treating before you spend a lot of money "fixing" it. Make sure any professional you work with, or who works with your child, has specific short-term goals that YOU understand. Not some jargon-filled list of developmental milestones, but real functional goals.

And above all else, remember you are the child's Mommy or Daddy or Nana or whatever. Your job is to play with your child every day. Down on the floor play, eye-to-eye, cheek-to-cheek; your job is not to complete a home program someone else thinks is critical. Children learn from the platform of the caring, trusting relationship they form with their parents. Everything else stems from that. So make that your priority … play and enjoy yourselves.

The Foundation's campaign to have SPD included in the DSM: Most people have no idea how important this is, Chynna. There are even people who are against this campaign. They don't want SPD to be a "mental disorder." But perhaps they don't realize the DSM includes learning disorders, motor disorders, communication disorders, social disorders, cognitive disorders and so on. We have to get a diagnostic code. Until then: a) our researchers will not get big NIH funding because SPD is "not a real diagnosis" and b) our families will have trouble getting reimbursement for therapies. It is a big deal, probably the most important legacy I can leave. Those who are "against" it will benefit as much as those who are neutral. But if everyone were to get behind the movement we would be unstoppable. Look what the parents of children with autism have accomplished! They are our role models. Each and every person can make a difference. We are up against an establishment that has deep roots, and prejudice dating back forty years. However, we have the ultimate weapon now; data. Data showing SPD is a valid disorder and that treatment works. (See www.SPDFoundation.net and click on "our library" to see articles on this topic).

Her thoughts on why getting the right diagnosis can be so difficult: Chynna, there are leapers and creepers. The doctors trained in the 70s, 80s, and 90s are right about one thing: the research on SPD conducted then was not compelling. In a way it's not their fault. It's hard to keep up. We have to have a sort of revolution to change thinking in this area. What Kuhn called equipoise. There has to be a shift in overall thought in the general public, or among professionals and parents who care about this area. We are like at a "tipping point."

Chances are pretty good that doctors and educators trained a few decades ago haven't seen the new research such as our two part series in Brain Research (a really good journal) showing brain differences in children who are typically developing compared to children with SPD. There are lots of other new compelling studies too. When I teach our mentees (professionals who come for our one week advanced educational experience) and after I review the top 10 new peer-reviewed publications on SPD, I tell them, next time someone says "There's no research … just say to them: oh that's just so 80s!"

Three ways to get on the right 'sensational' track: The first thing is to try to hook up with another parent who has been through this whose child is similar to yours. You will find that other parents are often the best source of information.

The second thing is to have a top-notch professional multi-disciplinary evaluation. Make sure the diagnosis is right, or the treatment may not work. Make sure that a qualified professional who also knows about (and believes in) SPD, rules out autism, ADHD, OCD, and other diagnoses. Or perhaps suggests a dual diagnoses (ADHD + SPD). Dual diagnoses are very common. But you have to get an accurate diagnosis to know what to do next.

Third, find a professional you can trust. One who is parent-centered, whose philosophy is to teach you everything they know. They might be an Occupational Therapist, a MD, a Speech/Language Pathologist, or someone else who can help YOU make the best decisions for your child and family. Make sure you know what is happening; do not give over decisions about your child to professionals. Find a professional who allows you to come into the treatment sessions, helps you to set realistic goals, and teaches you so that instead of a home program, you know what to do in real life situations. There is so much more, it's hard to write this all down! I have a good chapter on this in my book, *Sensational Kids*.

Pearls of wisdom for parents: There is hope and help for children with SPD and their families. You are not alone. Join us in our efforts to help you and others like you. Your efforts in our effort will come back manifold by way of learning how you can help your child. Sensational kids are just that ... sensational! Differently-abled! They are our future so lets get together and make a difference for them. Thank you for this opportunity to talk to parents, Chynna.

Lucy Jane Miller
April 26, 2012

About the Author

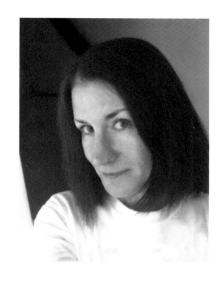

CHYNNA LAIRD – is a psychology major, freelance writer and author living in Edmonton, Alberta with her partner, Steve, and their three daughters [Jaimie (nine), Jordhan (seven), and Sophie (three)] and beautiful boy, Xander (five). Her passion is helping children and families living with Sensory Processing Disorder and other special needs.

You'll find her work in many online and in-print parenting, inspirational, Christian and writing publications in Canada, United States, Australia, and Britain. In addition, she's authored an award-winning children's book (*I'm Not Weird, I Have SPD*), two memoirs (the multi award-winning, *Not Just Spirited: A Mom's Sensational Journey With SPD* and *White Elephants*), a Young Adult novel (*Blackbird Flies*), an adult Suspense/Thriller (*Out of Sync*), and a Young Adult Suspense/Mystery/Paranormal/Sweet Romance (*Undertow*, to be released late summer/early fall 2012). She's also working on a sequel to *Not Just Spirited* called *Not Just Spirited: The Journey Continues* and a few other projects in the works for Middle Grade and Young Adult readers.

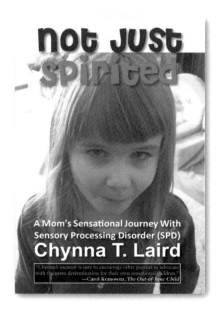

Please visit Chynna's Website at www.lilywolfwords.ca. To stay on top of her work, you can find her writing snippets at her author blog at www.chynna-laird-author.com, her SPD/special needs blog at www.the-gift-blog.com and her blog focusing on mental health and other issues at www.seethewhiteelephants.com.

CPSIA information can be obtained
at www.ICGtesting.com
Printed in the USA
LVIC06n2320300817
547049LV00015B/110